A Survivors Story

A Holistic Healing Journey Through Cancer

GENA BRADSHAW

BALBOA.PRESS

A DIVISION OF HAY HOUSE

Balboa Press books may be ordered through booksellers or by contacting:

Balboa Press
A Division of Hay House
1663 Liberty Drive
Bloomington, IN 47403
www.balboapress.com
844-682-1282

Because of the dynamic nature of the Internet, any web addresses or links contained in this book may have changed since publication and may no longer be valid. The views expressed in this work are solely those of the author and do not necessarily reflect the views of the publisher, and the publisher hereby disclaims any responsibility for them.

The author of this book does not dispense medical advice or prescribe the use of any technique as a form of treatment for physical, emotional, or medical problems without the advice of a physician, either directly or indirectly. The intent of the author is only to offer information of a general nature to help you in your quest for emotional and spiritual well-being. In the event you use any of the information in this book for yourself, which is your constitutional right, the author and the publisher assume no responsibility for your actions.

Any people depicted in stock imagery provided by Getty Images are models, and such images are being used for illustrative purposes only. Certain stock imagery © Getty Images.

Print information available on the last page.

ISBN: 978-1-9822-7760-4 (sc)
ISBN: 978-1-9822-7761-1 (e)

Balboa Press rev. date: 01/10/2022

CONTENTS

I would like to thank my incredibly loving and supportive family and friends, especially my parents. Without you all and faith, I could not have achieved this. Teamwork makes the dream work. And to all my cancer fighters and survivors I write this for you. We each go through our own journey but collectively know we are in this together. This is for you all.

I would also graciously love to thank the Cohen family, thank you for your help when our family was in need.

In Loving Memory of Stephanie Bradshaw

Everyone you encounter has some connection to cancer. Whether they suffered themselves or knew someone going through something so tragic. Cancer is the second leading cause of death in America. Why? How can something spread so quickly and cause overall life or death experience in the blink of an eye? These are the questions we may ask ourselves on a day-to-day basis. At 28 years old, I am a two-time cancer survivor, a pediatric and young adult survivor. My goal is to create less stigma around the word cancer and a better understanding of how lifestyle, mindset, and holistic health can play a big-time role. I hope my story will inspire others to take ownership of their health. Let's begin.

FOREWORD BY EUGENIA BRADSHAW

As I write this forward for my daughter Gena, I have immense feelings of pride and admiration. Eugenia Bradshaw, Gena for short was born on June 27, 1993, she is the oldest of five. Fast forward three and a half years, this is where her cancer journey began. She was three and a half and had her two brothers, Nicholas two years old and Raffaele two months old when she was diagnosed with leukemia, that's when it all changed.

From the beginning she was an active, healthy, happy out going child who had tons of energy. She had a spirit of adventure and loved the outdoors. Even through her battle with leukemia she loved to go to the beach, eat good food and play. There were days in the hospital where she could barely move and was so sick, but she would force herself to go to the playroom and try and have some fun. This battle went on for almost three years then another two of continued testing to make sure she was out of the woods.

By the time she was done with her treatment and testing period she had a new sister Anna Lieza. As a family we were very active and loved to cook and eat good food. Her love of a healthy lifestyle began and continues to this day. Growing up in a large Italian family with three boys, Anthony Tucker the youngest was born when Gena was eight, she was always competing with them. My husband and I were in the health and fitness business, so she took an interest at a young age. She would come to group training or team training sessions and jump right in to help. She loved to move and competition. When she started high school, I suggested she tryout for the cross-country team, she did but wasn't fond of it. She then continued with track and field and discovered a talent for sprinting and throwing the javelin, (which was encouraged by Ed Kilkelly an amazing man and coach who was a mentor to me). This led her to become a collegiate student-athlete at Ithaca College. She had no hesitation in deciding her major of exercise science and continued her journey. During her junior year she finds out that she had a 4cm growth in her neck. It turns out to be thyroid cancer…after her diagnosis she says, "great I had cancer twice." This was also the end of her junior year but was insistent on finishing her season and her finals, instead of bringing her down it made her stronger. She was determined to get over it and move on.

After college she immersed herself in the field and knew this was her path in life. She empowered herself with knowledge about fitness, nutrition, and overall wellness. She was determined to control all the things she could as far as her own health and help others do the same as part of her journey. As a mom I sat back and watched as my daughter went through these different phases in her life to get her where she is today. This is not to say we didn't battle along the way, we did, and but this was part of the journey.

When Gena told me she wanted to write a book about cancer my first thought was, I hope it doesn't bring her back to all that stress and fear and bring up all those emotions. As a parent the last thing you want is for your child to suffer. What I didn't realize was that it is part of her journey to heal and help others. She has gone through so much as a child, teenager and young adult and she figured out ways to deal with each stage. After reading her book I was happy that she remembered all the support and love that surrounded her and although the fear was there, she as a child wasn't sure why she was scared but she knew she was loved. She talks about how she felt as a child being diagnosed with cancer and not understanding things but feeling the love and support of her family. She explains how she felt when her grandmother, Stephanie was diagnosed and lost her battle with cancer when she was in high school and how that affected her. As parents we must understand children have feelings of fear and anxiety but don't know why. It's our job to comfort, communicate and hug them.

When Gena was in the thick of her treatment at times it was difficult to walk, she would get bad headaches and bone pain from the chemo. I knew she loved to be outside, and it was important for her to get fresh air and try and move. One day she wanted to go outside, and I would take a stroller with me in case she got too weak. We started on our walk on a beautiful sunny day and within minutes she was struggling. I reached over to pick her up and put her in the stroller, but she got mad and said NO, I want to walk. This is GENA determined and a fighter. When she started high school, she told me she was going to try out for the lacrosse team. If you know Long Island you know these kids are given lax sticks when they are three years old and have been playing for years before they get to high school. Gena was unable to do any of that because of treatment and a weak immune system. When she told me she was going to try out my first thought was…. oh no, I knew she wouldn't have the skill because she never played on an organized team. I knew she was athletic but that wasn't going to be enough. I kept my mouth shut and encouraged her to try, she got cut and came home shed some tears and said the girls were mean. Instead of shying away from athletics she went full steam ahead and never looked back. She thrives on a challenge, and it adds fuel to her fire.

She talks about how she felt when she was diagnosed as a junior in college, a fear she had been living with all those years. How she had to put up a brave front being the tough girl just to survive, (that's probably when we did most of our arguing). All of what she has experienced has given her the strength to be who she is today. She takes us through the different stages and what she has learned and gives us information to help us all be a better version of ourselves. We learn the importance of movement, mindset, support systems, and food to help us heal. She goes on to say how giving back is now part of her journey to continue to heal and living her best life. Gena's journey will help anyone going through stress, illness and uncertainty and teach us how to control what we can control and realize the importance of a positive mindset. To say I am proud of her is an understatement, I sit back and watch as my daughter continues her journey of health, wellness and happiness and teaches others to do the same. I feel blessed and thankful to learn and draw strength from you.

LOVE, MOM AND POP and *Keep Being You*!

INTRODUCTION

I am a two- time cancer survivor that was led into the health, fitness, and wellness industry at a young age and really brought my life full circle. Owning your health and wellbeing is so important, I want to share that knowledge and my experience with others to teach them and show there's hope. If you don't have your health, you don't have anything. I have created and provided some tips, tricks, tools and strategies regarding health, fitness, and wellness to optimize your lifestyle and peace of mind.

My hope is that everyone can learn about leading a healthy lifestyle, no matter where you are in life, what disease or diagnosis you have. It is all about a positive support system, awareness, mindset, resiliency, and determination. The mindset you have throughout your journey is 99% of the battle. It is imperative to create an internal awareness of healing and self-love while going through adversity and illness. As well as being proactive and preventative in teaching our youth while they can learn healthy habits, so that maybe we can avoid illness and or disease down the road. The way we think, fuel, and move our body is crucial, we may be predisposed to genetics, but it is the way we live our lives that pulls the trigger.

CHAPTER 1

THE BEGINNING

"God chooses his strongest soldiers for the toughest battles"

I was born in New York City, my parents and I lived in an apartment on the upper east side. My parents, Tucker and Eugenia Bradshaw were both dominant in the health and fitness industry, serious triathletes, business owners, and living a healthy lifestyle. They practiced what they preached and continue to every day. When I was one year old, we moved out of the city and to Port Washington, Long Island, the city became too expensive to raise a family. My parents were both commuting and working in the city at the time, continuing to grow our family fitness business, Bradshaw Personal Fitness. They also knew they wanted more kids and that would be difficult to afford in the city.

Now fast forward to me at age three and a half, my mom had my two-year-old brother, Nicholas and my two-month-old brother, Raffaele. It was around Christmas time, and I had been sick for a few weeks. I was very pale, had an ongoing cold that had gone into my chest and had to be put on prednisone. My mom had been taking me back and forth to the doctor, but he didn't seem to be alarmed. It was just after Christmas, and I had been sick for almost six weeks. We just moved into our new house; we were staying at my grandparents' house while work was being done on the house. It was now just after New Year, and I still wasn't feeling well. I didn't want to walk, coughing all the time, and as my mom said, pale as a ghost and had petechiae, (small bruising). She told me if she knew then what she knew now it would have been obvious to her. My mom once again went back and insisted on blood work. The doctor called her back and told her to come in so he could go over the results. He immediately sent my mom over to the Schneider's Children's Hospital, (now Cohen's Medical Center) although she had no idea what was about to unfold and what her daughter was about to go through. When she got to the hospital her brother met her there, and they immediately did a bone marrow aspiration from my hip. There was no anesthesia and my mom had to help hold her three-and-a-half-year-old daughter while they stuck what she described as a corkscrew into her young daughters' hip. From there they took her into a room with me on her lap, my uncle sitting next to her and about five other doctors sitting in a circle… The doctor said, "Your daughter has Leukemia and needs medical attention immediately." She said she heard nothing else after that and just looked at her brother in disbelief and wanted to collapse.

I asked my mom later on in life what her reaction was in that moment she said, "time stopped, everything just went blank, I couldn't process the information. The number one priority was to take care of you." I was then immediately admitted to the hospital for surgery for a mediport to administer chemotherapy, blood transfusions, x-rays, chemotherapy, and countless other medical treatments. This is where my cancer journey begins. I was diagnosed with Acute Lymphoblastic Leukemia. Small yet mighty is what the doctors and nurses used to say, they really did make the process a bit better. I remember my Oncologist, Janie, I thought she was the coolest. A very calm, funny, and passionate woman and she cared, I knew she cared. I can vividly remember getting finger pricks (which I would throw an absolute fit every time), blood work, constant monitoring my vitals, spinal taps, chemotherapy, the combative nature after getting "sleepy medicine," but most of all the playroom, our IV pole races down the hallway, and the clown visits. I can still remember one clown in particular, Therese, she attended my fifth birthday party and made balloon animals for all the kids. My absolute favorite part though was that my grandfather, who owned an Italian restaurant at the time in Westbury, Long Island, would cook me fresh homemade meals and bring it to the hospital, EVERYDAY. To this day he will say, "the food healed her."

What my little body and other pediatric patients went through is enough to kill a horse. The treatment and protocol that was used at the time (and still is evolving) was prescribed to adult cancer patients, it is like splitting an aspirin in half and giving it to a child. I lost all of my hair and since I was also on steroids, I had what one would call a "moon face" I was looking quite chunky. I remember feeling very much alone, isolated, angry, sad, abandoned, scared at such a young age. Having to fight for my life and the effect it has made on me today. According to Leukemia and Lymphoma Society research, 80% of pediatric cancer patients that survive can end up being diagnosed with another form of cancer or illness down the road. I am part of this statistic.

The Treatments I received:

Chemotherapy
Doxorubicin
Daunorubicin
Cyclophosphamide
Prednisone
Dexamethasone
Methotrexate
Cytarabine
Mercaptopurine
Thioguanine
Asparaginase
Vincristine
Intrathecal Methotrexate

Surgery
Mediport Insertion and Removal

Chemotherapy is extremely toxic and expensive. "In 2017, one 6mg Neulasta (type of chemo) injection cost between $5,000 and $7,000." (1) Not only does chemotherapy kill cancer cells, but it also kills all your healthy cells, completely wiping out your bodies defense mechanism. It specifically goes into the bone marrow where blood cells are manufactured and proliferated. If it gets to a point where the body cannot clot, the patient is at risk of bleeding to death. What happens when they must haul chemotherapy, or the body isn't receptive to it? The doctors are at a loss and so are you. There are no other alternatives being given in hospitals once this happens. This is where alternative and holistic medicine must come into play (which will be discussed in later chapters).

At Schneider's, which was a couple of years of a long and hard battle, my dad was working in NYC, came back to the hospital overnight, sleepless nights, then would go back to work in the city by 5am on repeat for a little over two years. My mom stopped working, committed to taking care of me and what was now three kids at the time. Almost losing their home. Truly I do not know how my parents did it. They are angels and never gave up. When adversity struck, they prevailed, were resilient, had faith, kept their health to the best of their ability, and we had the most incredible support system you could ask for. Yes, I went through some serious suffering, but I truly commend my family for having faith and keeping me alive. The stress on the family was enough to rip us apart, it only brought us closer.

During this time, we were involved in many non-profit organizations and fundraisers to help raise money for my family to survive, and to find a cure for cancer, specifically pediatric cancer. Team and Training, Leukemia and Lymphoma Society, Schneider's Children's Medical Foundation, Light the Night, The Jell-O Jump (this was my personal favorite), Cohen's Children's Medical Center, the list goes on. It is amazing to think back at all the incredible moments we shared as a family attending and participating in those fundraisers even going through one of the most difficult adversities. We also made so many friends along the way, one of our family friends to this day was in treatment the same time I was. My parents and parents of another pediatric cancer survivor, Nicole, (who is also a two-time cancer survivor), are best friends to this day. Our families being extremely close knit, we all participate in the cancer community together. Talk about full circle.

Out of all, if not most of the pediatric cancer patients, Nicole and I were the very few to survive in our group. While in the hospital, there was a clinical trial with new treatment to potentially cure us or at least try because at this point nothing else was working, all of us near death. I have personally faced death. I was the only one that wasn't allowed in the clinical trial due to prior protocol that I did not meet. Nicole was admitted into the trial, and ended up relapsing with Leukemia, as close to death as you could be. Literally planning her funeral. Thank God, Nicole survived. However, she became physically disabled, the neurotoxins from the chemotherapy and treatments caused permanent motor skill disability; speaking slowly, writing slowly, walking slowly, in need of assistance to perform daily life activities. However, Nicole is a total Rockstar and has continued her journey to help others that have suffered similarly.

There are many repercussions from receiving such intense drugs at such a young age. I was told that I have "chemo brain" which can affect the left side of the brain. Really all that affected me was being able to deal with numbers and math in my head, I need fingers or a calculator. However, the doctors did tell my parents that down the road I could potentially develop another form of cancer, which did happen to me at age 20.

To have cancer as a child is unbearable, let alone beyond comprehension, and the two words shouldn't co-exist. I wonder from time to time what caused me to be diagnosed with cancer. During my research on the topic of pediatric cancer, and what I discuss in this book, environment, virus, and carcinogens seem to destabilize DNA and can cause cancer (more on the topic later in the book). What could I have been exposed to and these other children? My mom has mentioned how her and my dad, and the other parents would chat about why this happened to their child. Interestingly, there was a trend around most of the kids receiving the MMR booster. When mentioned to the oncologist her response, "Most kids are diagnosed at this age when they get their shots, and it is just a coincidence." This should make us all question and think about what goes into children's bodies.

Although treatment for pediatric cancer must and needs to change. There are other ways we can ALL take control of our health. We must look at our daily habits and lifestyle, if you lead a toxic lifestyle, such as, eating poorly, sedentary most of the time, toxic people surrounding you, creating negative thoughts and emotions, stress constantly, lack sleep, using highly toxic products daily, lack of self-love, chances are quite high that you can develop heart disease, cancer, diabetes, autoimmune disease, etc. Let's review the basics.

What is chronic disease? It is a condition that lasts for one year or more, generally incurable, is usually a long-term behavioral problem, requires ongoing medical attention and limits a person's ability for normal daily activities. Heart disease, high blood pressure, asthma, cancer, and diabetes are often preventable and manageable with early detection, exercise, and improved diet. While adults are living longer, statistics show that chronic disease is the leading cause of death and disability in the United States. According to the CDC, almost 45% of the population has at least one chronic disease, and 75% of all health care costs goes to treat these conditions. (4)

As a society we consume high amounts of processed food, not enough whole grains, fruit, and vegetables, spend hours watching TV and video games, not nearly enough exercise, recreational activities, or sports and have easy access to tobacco. The Center for Disease Control and Prevention estimates that making massive changes to these three major risk factors, poor diet, inactivity and smoking would reduce heart disease, stroke and diabetes by almost 80%, and almost 40% of cancer patients. Prevention needs to continue with the work of Public Health Organizations educating about health and wellness within communities. Schools and hospitals having healthy options for the youth and sickly. Physicians being more proactive with their patients promoting how important a healthier lifestyle is, and consulting with health and fitness professionals regarding nutrition, exercise, and smoking programs. If we don't control this epidemic, over 50% population will be affected by 2025. (4)

Some things you can do to control and own your health:

- Exercise and daily movement
- Nourish your body with whole, fresh foods

- Hydrate with water
- Rest and recovery
- Stress and energy management
- Sleep, this is VERY important
- Do things you enjoy, love and have fun!

This may seem overwhelming; however, you can control ALL these variables with discipline, motivation, and the proper guidance. Throughout this book we will break down physical health, nutritional health, the brain, and how emotions and stress can in fact create disease.

CHAPTER 2

MY JOURNEY AS A CANCER SURVIVOR

"Never look back you are not going that way"

Fun fact I am the oldest of five siblings. We have a very big, close-knit family, a lot of cousins, we were always playing outdoors, hanging out and involved in sports together (still do). Growing up my siblings and I were involved in every sport imaginable. We are so grateful to our parents for getting us involved and most importantly keeping us involved. As a child though, I was a late bloomer because of being sick. Left behind in school as well, my parents placed me into a small Quaker school so I could interact with other kids, learn, and still be cautious of building my immune system back up. It is funny because when I was younger, I knew I was different, I just didn't know why or how. Even at a young age I couldn't comprehend what I had gone through and how traumatizing it was, I guess I thought everyone goes through that kind of pain and suffering. I started playing sports later in life, however my parents kept me involved in dance, which helped develop my motor skills (so smart on their part). Eventually by age six I was able to participate in sports. Where my other journey beings.

Entering into middle school I was completely acclimated to others and able to handle the workload. Although I had a tutor my entire life for math, which it is what it is, I used to be embarrassed about it but now I just say, "that is what calculators are for." Plus, I have yet to use the Pythagorean theorem anywhere at any point in the real world. Personally, I am a very sociable individual, I love engaging with others, the social aspect for school was great. I also developed a talent within sports. Ironically enough it led me to track and field, which also comes full circle, I had others running for me trying to raise money for my survival and now here I am running, competing, and coaching others on my own.

The opportunities to engage with others, listen to their stories, be an inspiration was a lot for me to handle. I couldn't comprehend it and unknowingly very emotionally draining. But I knew I had to do it to help heal myself and others. At age 13, I had the opportunity to be the speaker for the Children's Medical Foundation, where I met George Ross from the Apprentice. He was super cool. I got a great vibe from him; I specifically remember his super grandiose smile and powerful handshake. Truthfully, I had no idea what was going on, I kind of just did it, I don't remember being terribly nervous to speak in front of a couple hundred businessmen and women, including celebrities.

At age 16, my mom had graciously offered me up to speak at another fundraiser for Schneider's Children's Hospital at Cipriani Wall Street in NYC. She lied to me and said, "it is exactly like the last speaking event you did, only a couple hundred people." Well, I walk in and to my left is a ginormous stage and around the venue were five monster plasma screens that my face would be plastered on. This time I was so nervous I had to be carried into the venue and I was shaking. I told my mom, "Oh I'm not doing that, there is no way." She stares me dead in the eyes and says, "yes you are you have no choice put on your big girl pants, we are here, and this is happening." I had been working with my aunt to help me put together a speech, which I felt pretty confident in, but you put a 16-year-old girl on stage with monster screens plastering her face and you bet some insecurities come up. Suddenly, I forgot what I was going to say, I thought I was going to vomit everywhere. To be honest, I remember being on stage for a second, but everything went black. I rose to the occasion and apparently to my dismay gave an impeccable speech and a standing ovation. I met Ray Romano, Elvis Costello, and Melania Trump. We raised over 1 million dollars that night, and I am beyond thankful to my parents for pushing me to do something bigger than myself.

My track and field career all started at our local catholic all girls high school, Sacred Heart Academy (which I did not enjoy at the time, however, appreciate so much later in life). While attending, I met one of the most influential coaches of my life and he put me onto the path of track and field (besides my mom). The two years I attended that school, I developed great learning habits, life learning skills and I learned how to throw the javelin. My coach Ed Kilkelly scouted me out (rest his soul), he heard from my older cousins (who also attended SHA) that I had played softball for a little and had an arm. I knew I didn't want to continue with my softball career into high school, so I opted for track and field. My coach comes up to me and says, "Bradshaw! I heard you got an arm; I want you to try out for the track and field team and throw the javelin." I said, "Throw what?" Coach Kilkelly said, be at practice tomorrow and I will show you. From that point on it has been my love and passion. A little background on the javelin, this is literally a spear that you throw as far as you can and one of the highest scoring points in track and field. This event dates to ancient Greece time, it is one of the original sports and events.

During my two years at Sacred Heart Academy, tragedy struck, and my grandmother was diagnosed with melanoma. She was such a vivacious woman. While she was going through this, receiving treatment, she looked more and more sickly. I truly did not understand the severity of it, it didn't register to me that she had cancer. She never wanted us to see or know her pain. We were extremely close; she was the best human being God gifted this earth with. She lost her battle October 7th, 2009. This was devasting to process as a teenage girl and thinking, "here I had cancer and yet I survived, and she did not, since I had cancer no one else in my family should have to suffer." I believe subconsciously that moment triggered something in me, and I started to live in fear of getting cancer again or it affects someone I love. After two years I decided I needed to leave the all-girls school, so I transferred and attended another co-ed catholic high school in Long Island, St. Anthony's. Where this furthered my career in track and field.

Well, I became advanced and qualified enough to earn some scholarship money onto college and continue running and throwing at Ithaca College. This is also a full circle moment because my dad also attended Ithaca and was on the national championship football team. Technically I was a legacy. What did I decide to study? Exercise Science. Once again full circle moment. I knew I would never be behind a desk; I needed to move and live a healthy lifestyle. While my time at Ithaca, which was an incredible experience, alas adversity struck my junior year. One day, I had a very bad migraine (which I suffer from time to time), I went to the health center. I explained my pain and how maybe it could potentially be a sinus infection. The doctor starts to feel my lymph nodes in my neck, and I felt her pause and feel around my neck investigating the area. I had a feeling she noticed something. Never did I think it would be cancer. The doctor says, "I don't like what I am feeling by your thyroid." The first thought in my head… "what the hell does that even mean?" She then proceeds to explain about the main hormonal gland in our body, it is a very important regulator within our system. I asked what the next step would be. The doctor tells me that I need to book an appointment with the local ENT asap, which I did. I also did not mention any of this going on to anyone, not my coach, not even my family. I didn't really think much of it, I was kind of nervous, but I never thought that I would ever be diagnosed with cancer again, I just did what I had to do.

I ordered a cab and headed to the local ENT in Ithaca, New York. Once the appointment was finished, the doctor suggested that I get a biopsy at Cayuga Medical Center. I made that appointment and headed over to the medical center a day later. This all went on within the last two weeks of my junior year, where I was studying for finals, and training for our state championship meet that I had qualified for. The technician told me that it was a thyroid nodule, a hard lump in the thyroid, when he tested the slides, it seemed benign, however it needed to be removed soon and needed further testing. Fun fact the thyroid cells and cancer cells look extremely similar so sometimes you just can't tell. This nodule was sticking out of my neck and was 4cm big. I was lifting and training hard, so I thought it was muscular. Talk about neglecting my own body and not even realizing that this was a potential threat to my health. Finally, I called my parents and broke the news. I expected a totally freak out and that is what I got. I did not tell my coach at this point because I wanted to finish up school and the track season. What did my mom do? She called my coach. However, everyone was very helpful and receptive in the process. But how is anyone really supposed to act? The only thing that can be done is support that person emotionally and assist in any helping hand. While I was preparing for competition, my mom was making phone calls and was put in touch with two doctors that specialize in the thyroid.

Once I finished up with school and competing, which I ended up hitting a personal record in the javelin and 100m/200m sprint and a 3.8 GPA, I had scheduled appointments to meet with doctors who would complete my surgery. I met two different doctors, one had stated that they may have to remove my entire thyroid, be on medication for the rest of my life and potentially have to take radioactive iodine and that the other doctor I had been looking into he actually studied under. The other doctor told me that they would remove only half of my thyroid because it was encapsulated, no medication and no radioactive iodine. You can bet your bottom dollar that I chose the second doctor who is the number one thyroid surgeon in the world and was located at Memorial Sloane Kettering in NYC. P.S. prior to my surgery I booked a trip to Florida to live my best life, visit family, and I ended up doing the flying hydro board in the Fort Lauderdale Intercoastal I was above water, and it was the most peaceful, exhilarating feeling. That is when I knew all would be okay.

June 2nd, 2014, I went in for surgery at Memorial Sloane Kettering in NYC (right before my 21st birthday). I had a sinus infection going into it (probably because I was subconsciously stressing and had just come off of a stressful junior year). I couldn't eat prior to the surgery because of the anesthesia, I felt absolutely terrible. I remember walking down the hallway finally going into surgery, and I said, "let's get this fucking shit over with." Everyone laughed of course. To be honest I had no clue what to expect even speaking with the doctor prior to the surgery, Dr. Shaha, mentioned that my voice could change. I said, "what do you mean, I could have a different voice?!" He explained how the nodule was very close to my vocal cords and could potentially change my voice. Well thank goodness he was wrong, and it did not, it was slightly raspier post-surgery, but it ended up going back to normal. He also said to me that he doesn't believe at all that it was cancerous, so of course I wasn't worried, nor did I have any thought in my mind that it would end up being thyroid cancer. Post-surgery was honestly such a painful process and mentally challenging for me, I still didn't know that it was thyroid cancer until about a month or so post-surgery. I remember not being able to move my neck, nauseas all the time, couldn't eat food (which was the most upsetting for me because I LOVE food), I couldn't breathe, it was just awful, and I wouldn't wish that on my worst enemy.

Now this is interesting, I must mention that when tragedy strikes, how we cope with emotion and stress can trigger a physiological response on a cellular level, which you will learn in the coming chapters. My doctor mentioned to me that this nodule may have been growing since the age of 14 or 15, nodules on the thyroid are very slow growing. After doing my research, I have learned your inner world and how you internalize stress and emotion play a big role in illness and disease. The tragedy of my grandmother passing away from cancer when I was 14 years old and how I was coping internally may have triggered a response and it was a perfect storm. Also in Chinese herbal medicine, which you will also learn in the coming chapters, personality traits, environment and our emotions are directly correlated to how physical illness, disease, and injury can manifest.

In terms of coping, I had the most amazing support system that I could ever ask for, if I didn't have that I don't know how I would have been able to get through such a challenging and sad time in my life. Death was not an option for me, I felt that I had so much more to do and accomplish. I thank God every day for my mindset and my health. Slowly but surely, I started to move, walk, eat healing foods to nourish my mind and body and just laugh. Not to mention, I took the summer to recover and train, I went back to Ithaca, finished up my senior year, competed the whole year, hit a personal record and finished up my degree in four years. I must say, I am badass. I had to have such a positive mindset and awareness all would be okay, or I don't believe I would have healed the way I did. Which leads me into why I wanted to write this book. I believe our bodies and minds are made to heal themselves and fight off disease when nourished and moved properly. We must battle too many harsh chemicals in our environment, water, foods, and products. That can be too much for the immune system, pair that with self-hatred and fear, in turn can cause chronic illness and disease. Your body will tell you when something is wrong, you just can't ignore the warning signs.

CHAPTER 3

THE HISTORY AND
IMPACT OF CANCER

"The ability to learn is the most important quality a leader can have."
-Sheryl Sandberg

To understand the severity of where the cancer industry is right now, we need to review the history. The "war on cancer" was declared in 1971, by President Nixon. He signed into law the National Cancer Act, which allocated 1.5 billion dollars for cancer research. How have we done you ask? According to World Health Organization, released in 2014, predicted new cancer cases will rise from estimated 14 million annually in 2012 to 22 million within two decades. Cancer deaths are predicted to rise from 8.2 million a year to 13 million. (1) If that doesn't raise your eyebrows, not sure what would. The cancer industry is worth billions, in 2014 the National Cancer Institute stated that medical costs of cancer care were $125 billion with a projected increase to $173 billion by 2020.

What this shows is that the cancer industry has lost its way, though it has brought a tremendous amount of knowledge regarding this disease. The industry has put all its eggs in one basket, they are only allowing big pharma to play a role in this "war." What about holistic and natural therapy healing? Why are we not talking about lifestyle, diet, movement, herbal and medicinal plants for healing? Which by the way most is of no cost, nature offers us plenty of healing modalities within plants and in their natural state, why are we not taking advantage?

Simple, money and power. "The cost of cancer drugs has skyrocketed in the last fifteen years. The average cancer drugs price for approximately one year of therapy was less than $10,000 before 2000. By 2005, it had increased from $30,000 to $50,000. In 2012, twelve of thirteen new drugs approved for cancer indications were priced above $100,000 per year of therapy. With typical out of pocket expenses at 20 to 30 percent, many patients (approximately 10 to 20 percent) are priced out and may decide not to take the treatment or may compromise significantly on the treatment plan." (1) Not only that but let's talk about pediatric cancer, according to Leukemia and Lymphoma Society research, 80% of pediatric cancer survivors end up with a chronic illness or another form of cancer post treatment down the road. According to MaxLove Project, a non-profit organization geared towards pediatric cancer, stated that less than 4% of U.S. government's total funding for cancer research is dedicated to childhood cancers each year. So again, I ask, why is that? We have put billions and billions of dollars into cancer research and there is no cure?

People are craving natural remedies that are effective and affordable, and there are however, it is being pushed off the shelves because it offers no "kick back" to any parties involved. Nearly 58% of individuals who consume dietary supplements report they do so for the prevention or treatment of cancer. (1) I have been doing a lot of research over the years through my own journey of being the healthiest version of myself and I have come across some natural remedies right out of the book, *Winning the War on Cancer* (which I use to this day). The Beljanski Foundation is dedicated to natural remedies to cure cancer. Here is what I have learned.

The work of Mirko Beljanski is extraordinary, he identified a new scientific way to look at cancer and treat it with natural ingredients and plants, proving its resiliency and can be most powerful when in combination of modern-day medicine. He developed four natural supplements that can benefit the cancer patient.

"Two of them (extracts of *Pao Pereira* and *Rauwolfia vomitoria*) have selective anticancer activity, meaning that they selectively damage cancer cells, but not normal cells. One of them (RNA fragments from nonpathogenic E.coli) is useful for stimulating all types of normal white blood cells and platelets, and is particularly beneficial for patients undergoing radiation and or chemotherapy. Finally, the last one, a specific extract from *Gingko Bilbo*, has been used as a nutritional supplement to help prevent abnormal scar tissue formation from radiation or surgery." (1)

More than a thousand clinical trials of dietary supplements are reported on *Clinicaltrials.gov*, yet the FDA has not approved any food or dietary supplement to prevent cancer, halt its growth, or prevent its recurrence. If certain foods provide healing, anti-cancer properties then why are they not approved or used in treatments? Such as green tea, pomegranate, lycopene, soy, mistletoe, vitamin C, D and, E, selenium, resveratrol as treatments. We will discuss nutrition and food in the coming chapter.

It is a bit disheartening to review this research knowing there are natural remedies and cures to help beat cancer and yet they are being halted or destroyed by big pharma because of money and politics. My mom used to give me certain supplements such as, acidophilus and fiber acid to help my stomach while I was undergoing chemotherapy. The nurses and doctors advised against, but she did it anyways. I thank her for that. Here was a typical day of treatment for me during my battle with Leukemia:

Vanco 6:30am

Imp 7:45am

Bactrim 8am

Acidophilus 11:30am

Fiber Acid

Vanco 1:30pm

Imp 1:30pm
Acidophilus 7:30pm
Bactrim 8:30pm
Vanco 9:30pm
Imp 10:30pm
Mouthcare 11:30am, 7:30pm

As a three-and-a-half-year-old, I was taking rounds of chemotherapy that was prescribed for adults. I think about how absolutely insane that is, according to Leukemia and Lymphoma Society research there has been only four approved drugs (as of 2021 now five) for pediatric cancer patients within the last 40 years. They are specifically working on another type of treatment, where they re-engineer the HIV virus to fight and attack only cancer cells, there has been success rate with this, this was developed by Dr. June.

Based off Mirko Beljanski's research with the natural remedies listed prior, he concludes that both pancreatic and ovarian cancers are often diagnosed late and develop drug resistance making it very difficult to treat. Since performing these studies on cells, then mice, the evidence was clear and revealed the following:

- The extracts are nontoxic to ordinary human cells
- The extracts have a selective effect against several lines of cancer cells
- The extracts work in synergy with chemotherapies
- Regarding the effect on ovarian cancer: the conclusion was that "In vivo, Pao Pereira alone suppressed tumor growth by 79 percent and decreased volume of ascites (the excess accumulation of fluid in the abdominal cavity) by 55 percent. When Pao Pereira was combined with Carboplatin (chemotherapy drug) tumor inhibition reached 97 percent" (1)

The evidence and research clearly indicate the combination of natural remedies and chemotherapy can co-exist and work together. The combination of both eastern and western medicine is POWERFUL, if we would be offering these natural remedies during treatments, giving patients healthy healing whole foods instead of processed and cancer feeding hospital foods, implementing movement, incorporating acupuncture, frequency sound healing, laughing, the survival rate would be much higher and not to mention their bodies would recover at a quicker rate with a much less risk of developing other types of cancers or illnesses down the road.

What exactly causes cancer? According to Mirko Beljanski, molecules can influence our DNA structures and some of these carcinogens can destabilize the DNA by breaking down the bonds, separating the two strands of the double helix. He proved that the primary difference between normal and cancer DNA lies in the increased opening between the two strands of the double helix, which leads to DNA destabilization. (1) That means there is a direct correlation to environmental carcinogens and the negative affect it has on our bodies and DNA. Now what is even more interesting is the number of carcinogens in all our home care, beauty care, foods, water, baby food, environmental products…

In *Clean Beauty Checklist* by In On Around You, Catherine, breaks down EVERY chemical that negatively affects our health and can predispose us to cancer, in fact, two-thirds of cancer diagnosis are due to environmental factors. Let's look:

Example: "Aluminum Compounds: aluminum chloride, aluminum chloralhydrate, alumina, magnesium aluminum silicate, aluminum starch, activated alumina, aluminum oxide, aluminum trichloride, trichloroaluminum" (2)

Why avoid it? It is potentially linked to bioaccumulation, breast cancer, Alzheimer's disease, and skin irritation. (2)

How is it used? In sweat and odor production, and as an anticaking agent, most found in antiperspirants. (2)

This is just the tip of the iceberg. We all use antiperspirants EVERYDAY.

An obvious, carcinogen is smoking tobacco products, which ironically enough the FDA stated it was safe for human consumption… According to Deepak Chopra, 30% of deaths in the U.S. are due to tobacco use. It can put a person at risk for up to 14 different types of cancer. Now the vapes have come into play, these smokeless tobacco products are responsible for 400,000 cases or oral cancer worldwide. (12)

How does cancer begin?

Cancer begins when a cell undergoes a mutation (which Mirko Belajnski has proven in his studies), one or more of its genes are damaged or lost. However, this doesn't happen overnight, there are different mutations that must happen before the cell becomes a cancer cell. Since time is a factor, we see this more so in older people because more time for mutations and exposures to carcinogens. (12)

The rate of division is what is concerning, it may be faster in some cancers but in all cancers the cells never stop dividing. Cancer is hundreds of different diseases. It originates in one area and can spread to different areas due to cell reproduction and tumor growth. It is like a race against time, just know there is **hope.** Genetics do play a role, but it is the way that you live your life, what you put into your body, on it and around it that can pull the trigger. Just think though, if you have the capability to turn genes on, then you also have the capability to turn them off (the ones that would negatively impact your health).

Cancerous tumors also shed cells into the bloodstream. "It's estimated that a 1cm tumor sheds more than a million cells into the circulatory system in just 24 hours." (12) I had to process that for myself because the nodule on my thyroid was 4cm large…Most of these cells are killed by cells of the immune system or die due to injury, but some may survive.

Think about how much our immune systems and bodies are hit with daily, it is quite alarming. You can seriously go down to even the candles you use in your home. The American standard diet, filled with chemicals, processed, sugary foods feed virus, illness, inflammation, and cancer, so why are we harming our bodies in this way? We need to be more aware of what we are ingesting, putting in and on our bodies, toxic environments/people, stress, energy, and self-love.

In the coming chapters I am going to break down the key components to living a healthier and happier life, even if you are struck with illness your body will fight for you, it's designed to, if you treat it properly. I want to share my knowledge with you all so that you can take back control of your health TODAY. The *"7 Gems of Mastery,"* is what my co-host Erica Suter and I came up with to help others take control of their lives again, we discuss them on our podcast, **Girls to Queens.** It is your given birth right to own your health and well-being, so do just that. (3)

Most wonder, why me? Why did I get cancer, what did I do wrong? As a child, I did nothing wrong to be diagnosed with cancer, a series of unfortunate events. As a young adult or adult being diagnosed, there are variables that play a role in your lifestyle for sure. Besides toxic environment, which is a given, after Erica and I came up with our *"7 Gems of Mastery,"* I came across in *Winning the War on Cancer,* by Sylvie Beljanski, her take on personality traits and the type of person she has noticed that is diagnosed with cancer. Our *"7 Gems of Mastery"* and what Sylvie had taken note of were practically identical. This was an ah-ha moment for me.

Girls to Queens Podcast: 7 Gems of Mastery

1. Purpose: what is your why?

2. Relationships: the quality of your relationships are the quality of your life.

3. Nutrition: how do you nourish and fuel your body?

4. Physical Health: daily movement, strength, and activity, be playful.

5. Emotional/Energy/Mental Health: energy, mood, motivation.

6. Sleep/Recovery/Stress Management

7. Leisure: travel, hobbies, fun, passions, playful. (3)

What Sylvie describes in, *Winning the War On Cancer,* is an observation in her cancer patients and their personality traits. Which goes hand in hand with the *"7*

Gems of Mastery." She has seen many patients over the last 28 years and has observed different personality traits in "cancer susceptible" individuals. These traits are as follows:

1) "Being highly conscientious, caring, dutiful, responsible, hardworking, and usually of above average intelligence.

2) Exhibits a strong tendency toward carrying other people's burdens and taking of extra obligations, often "worrying for others."

3) Having a deep-seated need to make others happy. Being a people please with a great need for approval.

4) Often lacking closeness with one or both parents, which sometimes, later in life, results in lack of closeness with spouse or others who would normally be close.

5) Harbors long suppressed toxic emotions, such as anger, resentment and or hostility. The cancer susceptible individual typically internalizes such emotions and has great difficulty expressing them.

6) Reacts adversely to stress, and often becomes unable to cope adequately with such stress. Usually experiences an especially damaging event about two years before the onset of detectable cancer. The patient is not able to cope with this traumatic event or series of events, which comes as a last straw on top of years of suppressed reactions to stress.

7) Has an inability to resolve deep seated emotional conflicts, usually beginning in childhood, often even unaware of their presence, as noted above, is the long-standing tendency to suppress toxic emotions, particularly anger." (1)

Taking note of that and realizing that most cancers are not caused by genetic defects suggests that in most cases we have the power to modify or eliminate most of the factors that lead to it (you can change how your body heals). The most common risk factor for cancer is chronic (long-term) inflammation in the body. Inflammation is a normal part of your body's immune system response to injury. Problems arise when that inflammation becomes chronic.

When there is chronic inflammation in the body, there is a chemical response. "These substances include cytokines enzymes and adhesion molecules. All of these various chemicals have been linked to the development of cancerous tumors, and chronic inflammation precedes tumor growth in most types of cancer." (15)

What do we know causes cancer and why? Obesity, smoking, alcohol, infectious agents, carcinogens in food, water, and in the environment, internal stress, and fear, have been shown to cause chronic inflammation in the body. The longer the inflammation continues, the greater the risk of cancer.

In Chapter 5, I will discuss further and the connection between food, personality traits and disease. What you can do TODAY to reverse the process and heal.

CHAPTER 4

MOVEMENT IS MEDICINE

"If you don't use it, you lose it"

God gave us bodies, vehicles, to MOVE and enjoy them freely. However, we must take care of our mind and bodies, it is a temple. When we are sedentary, we become stagnant, when that happens, things can start to manifest negatively in the body. Chronic inflammation can and will lead to dysfunction and or disease within the body, disrupting homeostasis, it is just a matter of when. Our current lifestyles and enhancement of technology has made all our lives EASY. However, it comes at a cost. Sitting down twelve hours out of your day behind a desk and a computer is not how the human body was designed. Prehistorically we had to walk miles on miles to travel, hunt for food, care for family, SURVIVE. Today, that survival mechanism isn't needed, unless in a circumstance where it is fight or flight and you are seriously in trouble and need to save your own life.

When we sit for just twenty minutes in poor posture, this negatively affects our minds and bodies. We enter what is called "creep" mode, our fascia which is like saran wrap covers our muscles. In poor posture our fascia then molds to this and causes disruption in breathing, maybe you experience pain in your neck or back, however this can be reversed. How you ask? MOVEMENT, another modality would be to foam roll. This is something that can reverse the effects of "creep." This modality creates movement of fluid throughout the system, when there is movement and flow, we feel better. Stagnation is what causes disruption to our systems. Foam rolling is a part of every single one of our client's exercise programming, whether they are an athlete or considered general population, they know it works and have experienced the benefits.

Let's discuss some health benefits of physical activity/exercise/movement (no matter, age, level, or gender):

- Reduce the risk of illness/disease (long term positive influence) (cancer, type 2 diabetes, Alzheimer's, dementia, heart disease, obesity)
- Increase in brain function/mental focus
- Energy boosting
- Longevity of quality life (5)

Overall optimal health creates homeostasis for your body within all physiological systems. Our bodies are constantly fighting disease, as I sit here writing this book my body is fighting disease, carcinogens, cancer cells, toxins, invaders to the body. We have so many defense systems that are just fighting for us. According to Dr. William Li, we have five different defense systems: our blood vessels, stem cells, gut microbiome, DNA, and our immune system. Just as little as twelve minutes a day of walking can improve the efficiency of all your bodies defense systems. However, the combination of both strength training and aerobic exercise are the most beneficial to overall health.

The number one leading risk for death is cardiovascular disease (CVD) which can be caused by hypertension (elevated blood pressure). The U.S. population holds 29% of people with hypertension. Just with baseline exercise and movement you can decrease that risk of developing CVD or hypertension significantly. In a research study, there was eight weeks of combined training of aerobic and strength training to combat the risk of hypertension or CVD. Not only did they see benefits in the group's overall health. They in fact did find that the combination of both aerobic and strength training was most beneficial than those who did aerobic or strength training alone. Movement is a key factor and should be used as a preventative measure to fight disease. We do not need to rely solely on pharmaceutical companies to prescribe medication when lifestyle modification is the most well-known way to help. (7)

A pattern that I have noticed being in the health and fitness industry for a decade, is that most people are stressed to the absolute max, lack daily movement, and do not know how to release/manage stress, emotions, and anxiety appropriately. Most of us are overworked, overstressed, overanxious, over literally everything. What I noticed was a pattern in human beings and society, the way we view life, and how we are just fighting to survive and get by, not thrive.

This in turn really hinders our health, a toxic environment is what leads to disease and illness, sometimes faster than we hoped. Knowing this, we continue to abuse, stress, and create a serious fight or flight mode for our bodies, internally. I was the Metabolic Specialist at Life Time Athletic for some time, I ran the submaximal and VO2 max testing, active and at rest. I noticed a similar pattern in the individuals I assessed.

While conducting these tests in an active state, it was executed on a treadmill, bike, erg, kettlebells, etc. depending on what modality the client utilized the most. While at rest, the client would be sitting comfortably in a chair and just breathing, not sleeping just resting. In both assessments, the individual was connected to a system called, smart leaf analyzer, where they would breathe into a mouthpiece and their CO_2 output would be analyzed through this system, as well as being hooked up to a heart rate monitor. This would test the metabolic systems and would show us the exact percentage the individual was utilizing carbohydrates and fats and what system they utilized the most. Based off this assessment, I then was able to gauge what type of training and nutritional style would be best suitable for them and their goals.

At certain intensity levels while active certain metabolic systems take over and run the show. For example, while we are at rest and just breathing, laying down, where our bodies are just functioning, you should be utilizing fat for fuel, this is the preferred energy source. The reason being is that as human beings we have more stored body fat, it is the healthiest way our bodies can function optimally, specifically less than 60% -70% of our intensity in energy expenditure. If our body is not able to utilize fat as a fuel source within that intensity range (also very much depends on the individual), then that can indicate the persons hormones, adrenaline and cortisol levels are too high and running the show. When that happens, the body chooses to utilize carbohydrates (glycogen) as a fuel source which is stored mostly in our muscles. This is not optimal; this means you are taking fuel from your muscles and most likely not replenishing that fuel source (insert poor eating habits) and basically running on empty. In turn the body is in chaos, thinking it is in survival mode and when that happens it completely throws your hormones and other physiological systems out of whack. Most individuals that exhibited this, exercised too much or not at all, overweight or underweight with no muscle tone, doing high intensity exercise more than 3x's per week putting their bodies into more of a fight or flight response, suffering from chronic illness, on medications, and living a very high stress/anxiety/fear filled life. Their heart rates at rest were usually very elevated even when just sitting breathing (one could argue that anticipatory factor plays a role).

The best example here is to compare this to your car. It is a machine, that runs on fuel source (well most cars now), if you are on dead empty gas and continue driving, what happens? The car starts to break down and sooner or later the car stops all together because it has no more fuel to keep going. That wear and tear is no good for the car and eventually can lead to problems. Well, our bodies are the same way, we are machines, and if not taken care of and fueled properly we can and will break down.

Chronic stress is not adaptive it is maladaptive states Dr. Joe Dispenza. "When we are living in survival mode and those hormones of stress like adrenaline and cortisol keep pumping through our body, we stay on high alert instead of returning to balance. When this imbalance is maintained for long term, chances are we are headed towards disease, because this long-term stress down regulates the healthy expressions of the gene. In fact, our bodies become so conditioned to this rush of chemicals that they become addicted to them. Our bodies actually crave them." (18)

When our hormones are out of whack it throws us into a spiral and negatively impacts our health. The sympathetic response, which would be fight or flight mode, triggers our hormones like cortisol, drives our heart rates up, increases internal stress, increases blood pressure, in turn can cause anxiety, fear, upset stomach, monkey mind, headaches, etc. What can we do about that you ask? MOVE, MOVE, MOVE! The evidence is as clear as day that movement is medicine.

There is such a clear link between obesity and cancer, in men it causes 24% of deaths and women 20% of deaths. Obesity is linked to many cancers, including cancers of the colon, breast, endometrium (uterine lining), esophagus, and kidneys. (12)

What about if you have cancer and want to exercise? MOVE!

Sara Mansfield, M.S., a certified cancer exercise trainer at Mayo Clinic Healthy Living Program, says that physical activity can help people before, during and after cancer treatments. It is so much more beneficial to your health to move during this time. The bounce back from the disease and treatment may be quicker if you exercise and move more. (6)

"When researchers reviewed 61 studies involving women with stage 2 breast cancer, they found that a combination of aerobic and resistance exercise was not only safe, but it also improved health outcomes. Other studies have found that exercise during treatment can change the tumor microenvironment and trigger stronger anti-tumor activity in your immune system. And very recent animal studies have found that exercise can lead to tumor reduction in rodents. Physical activity also helps you manage your weight, which is an important cancer risk factor." (6) What is so fascinating is that exercise and movement inhibit tumor growth. Even if you are overweight and you exercise there is still a positive effect, and it still lowers these cancer promoters.

This may seem overwhelming; however, you can control ALL these variables with discipline, motivation, and the proper guidance from a coach/trainer. What we can do as fitness professionals and coaches is to help: educate the people on how to exercise properly and efficiently based off their lifestyle/habits. How to nourish and fuel their bodies properly, manage stress, incorporate recovery, monitor sleep and hydrate with water often. There are many pieces to the puzzle in how we can help become healthy individuals and maintain that. Finding a knowledgeable health and fitness professional is key, often individuals will find coaches/trainers who really do more harm than good to their clients…choose wisely.

I am living proof that movement and exercise can heal you! I am so blessed to be a part of a family fitness business, we all practice what we preach, I cannot imagine myself doing anything different. There is beyond enough research out there to prove to you it is and even if you don't believe get out there and start moving yourself. I can bet you will feel way better than sitting around all day.

CHAPTER 5

FOOD IS FUEL

"Time and health are two precious assets we don't appreciate until they are depleted"
-Denis Waitley

The topic of food and its healing properties for the mind, body, and soul dates back centuries. Personally, my journey as a two-time cancer survivor was no easy ride, however my belief, research, and knowledge, has led me down a path of healing. You are what you eat, a very simple yet effective way of thinking, and played a HUGE role in my healing. Had I been eating McDonalds every day; I doubt I would have healed and survived cancer. Your health is vastly affected by what you ingest, which again can either feed the inflammation in your body, or stop it, the choice is yours. My path has led me to a place where the combination of simple, eastern traditional eating styles, patterns, and modern nutrition has saved my life and I hope to share that information with you.

In the United States, we view food just as food, to sustain living, to indulge in, and overeat. When in fact we are completely missing the boat. Whole foods contain tons of nutrients and minerals to sustain trillions of metabolic functions in the body as a whole. What you eat will either harm you or help you. In 1988, the Surgeon General acknowledged the value of a proper nutrition, "Fully two-thirds of all deaths are directly affected by improper diet, and poor eating habits play a large part in the nation's most common killers- coronary heart disease, stroke, atherosclerosis, diabetes, and some cancers."(8)

Food acts as a foundation medicine, which stems from our ancestors. Herbs, spices, and whole foods provide our medicine to heal. The American standard diet and western way isn't cutting it- genetically modified food, synthetic, pesticides, antibiotics, sugar, heavy metals, pollutants, refined white flour, junk food, hydrogenated oils the list goes on. My advice is to check out, do some research and more information at <u>ewg.org</u>.

Truthfully…it's killing us. According to research a study done in 2019 New England Journal of Medicine, stated that by 2030 some states will have obesity rates over 60%! Based off the research given in the previous chapter, that can increase risk to disease and illness. Also, according to the CDC, almost 45% of the population has at least one chronic disease. Those statistics are extremely eye opening. Unfortunately, most of us view this too late in the game, then you become discouraged, loop back into poor eating habits, become overwhelmed, and frankly just give up, until it's too late (oh and let's not forget what garbage the mainstream media feeds you). You can heal yourself; you just need to put in the work and **listen to thy self**.

Eastern Asian traditions really spoke to me when it came to my own healing and the connection to the body through food. If we can take the foundation from their culture and our western modern nutrition, we wouldn't depend on big pharma. "Thousands of years ago, master healers in China perceived a way to classify food and disease according to simple, easy and observed patterns: one eats cooling foods for overheated conditions, and warming foods are best for people who feel too cold. Detoxifying foods are for those who carry excess toxins, building foods are good for deficient persons." (8)

What this explains, we must view food as healing the individual based off their personality traits, how they carry/manage stress, how they handle their emotions, if they are sedentary, etc. Based on this holistic view you can prescribe, suggest, or eliminate certain food groups. Everything is in balance and harmony, that means certain foods can throw you in or out of balance.

Let's discuss cooking, this happens to be one of my favorite activities. Growing up in a big Italian family, food is seen as healing and filled with nutrients to sustain an optimal healthy life. Farm to table kind of lifestyle, homecooked meals every night, the family cooking together, sitting down and being mindful of eating and enjoying the food, culturally it shows love.

Knowing this, it is only right to go over the element of food preparation, most overlook this factor, in our society (Western), cooking is seen as an inconvenience, seen as a chore, overwhelming, the list goes on. What we fail to realize is that the preparation of your food sets the tone. Mixing certain food groups together in synchronization, making it come to life, more potent and bioavailable for our bodies to absorb and utilize nutrients. For example, in middle eastern countries they use turmeric as a spice in most of their cooking, if you add black pepper into the mix, it makes the anti-inflammatory property in turmeric 10x more potent. If you are not enjoying the process of cooking and putting love into your meals, it does play a role in the way your body processes the food. Are you eating fast? Are you mindful and grateful while eating your meal? Are you tasting your food? Are you on your phone the whole time or watching tv? Are you preparing your food in hydrogenated oils?

For example, in the Italian culture, lunch is our biggest meal, everyone sits down as a family and enjoys the meal in courses. A base to many of our meals is always extra virgin olive oil, the first press of the olives, the most beneficial good fat for overall health. A fun activity as a family, would be to learn about your nationality's dishes. What kind of herbs and spices are used as a base? What is their native home dish? Is this a plant-based diet, meat, carbohydrate, or fat predominance?

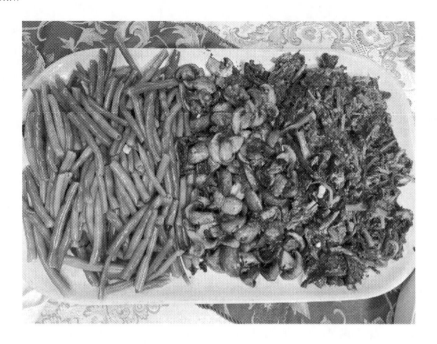

Let's discuss next where our food source is coming from. My absolute best advice would be to shop local grown, farm to table style. Fresh whole foods are best for our overall health, it all depends on where it is grown. When you go into a supermarket, most of the produce is shipped into our country, let's think about this. For example, avocado's, they are excellent for our overall health, they are considered a healthy fat. They are shipped over from California or Mexico. Which avocado would you choose if they looked identical? If you guessed California, that is what I would have guessed. The reason being is the shelf life, how long has the avocado been in travel, and how long has it been in the supermarket? These are the key factors we need to be aware of. When we shop locally and farm to table style, the soil may be richer and provide more nutrients in it, less pesticides if any, in season which means extra nutrients, and better tasting. Today's food, nutrients are diminished, although shopping smart, it all comes down to the source. Ironically in the United States, a land of the plenty-indeed excess- many people are highly deficient in minerals because of our food production and processing methods. As such, these deficiencies can lead to degenerative diseases. This is not surprising, what you feed your body, helps or harms.

Example: "Consider this grain before its milled into flour- "wheat berries." These whole-wheat seeds can comprise dozens of minerals and microminerals if grown in rich soil. They can contain immune-protective phytonutrients as well as vitamins and precious oils. In refining, as is done in the milling of wheat berries to obtain "white" flour used in common pastries, donuts, pastas, and breads, many of these nutrients are lost." (8)

Now, within that process these two most vital minerals for optimal body function are stripped during this process, they are selenium and magnesium. Most of the population suffers from everyday symptoms, such as headaches, backaches, fatigue, brain fog, etc.

Let's review some signs of mineral deficiencies:

- weak immunity
- allergies
- acne/rashes
- infections
- headache
- fatigue
- tooth decay
- brittle nails/hair
- lethargy
- abdominal cramps
- heart palpitations
- ringing in ears
- nauseas/vomiting
- dizziness
- pale skin
- low body temperature
- swollen tongue
- slow metabolism

- slow wound healing
- infertility
- memory problems

Interesting how everyday symptoms are signs of mineral deficiencies. I always refer out and advise a holistic or naturopathic doctor to dive further into if you have any nutrient/mineral deficiency. Is it possibly a cause as to why you are getting these everyday symptoms? Most women suffer from menstrual cramps, this can be a mineral deficiency in magnesium.

If we tie poor eating habits with personality traits and how you handle your emotions as a human being you will create an inner storm, which will manifest into physical form in your body, hence disease. How you live your life daily entirely impacts your health, it is a direct correlation. Leading a toxic lifestyle negatively impacts us. Relationships, eating, movement, sleep, hydration, leisure, and fun activity, it ALL matters. In the book, *Winning The War On Cancer*, Sylvie Beljanski, states her observation on dealing with cancer patients (which I stated in Chapter 3), it is also correlated to other illnesses and your body may manifest this in different ways physically.

This information will get your gears turning. Consider how you are living your life daily, really reflect on it. Every single human being is different, you know what your body needs, you just need to listen.

In terms of knowing thy self, let's review what we know as the personality traits, emotions, and how those connect. In Ancient Chinese Medicine, the five elements are the basis of life: wood, fire, earth, metal, water. All aspects that encompass these elements are patterns, internal organs, emotions, body parts, and environment. Viewing the whole individual, not just as parts. Hippocrates said, "It is more important to know what kind of person has disease, than to know what kind of disease a person has."

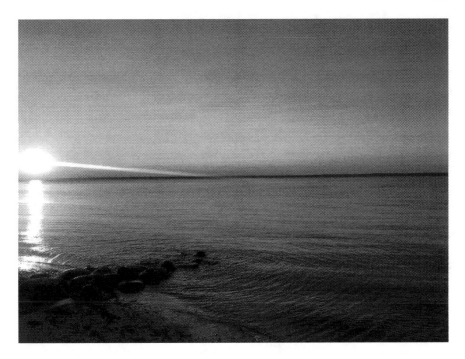

The Five Elements:

Wood element: Springtime, which means things are in bloom. Naturally we as human beings cleanse out the fats and extra storage from the wintertime. Which means our liver and gallbladder are seriously put to work. The types of foods that are best for this time of the year:

- o Young plants
- o Fresh greens
- o Sprouts
- o Immature wheat
- o Basil, fennel, marjoram, rosemary (8)

Fire Element: Summertime, this is a time of creativity and growth. Our bodies need bright colored fruits and vegetables, create beautiful meals. Sweating during the summer is normal and so we lose minerals and oils this way. Surprisingly, the combination of the heat and eating too many cold foods will make our digestion organs contract, therefore it holds in sweat and heat, interfering with digestion. The types of foods that are best for this time of the year:

- o Salads
- o Sprouts (mung, alfalfa)
- o Fruit (watermelon, lime, lemon, apples)
- o Cucumbers
- o Leaf teas

Our hearts and small intestine are the organs associated with this element. Dean Ornish, M.D., heart specialist at the University of California, stated "I think the mind is where the heart disease begins for many people." (8)

Earth Element: Late Summertime, this is a shorter period, the transition of warm weather to cooler weather of fall and winter. This element is represented by the spleen-pancreas, and stomach, the types of food best for those organs are:

- o Millet
- o Corn
- o Carrots
- o Cabbage
- o Garbanzo beans
- o Sweet potatoes/all types of potatoes
- o String beans
- o Yams
- o Sweet rice, amaranth
- o Peas
- o Chestnuts
- o Apricots, cantaloupe (8)

Metal Element: Autumn, this is the season of harvest and now the weather is cooler. The lungs and colon represent this element, which makes sense considering most of us suffer from allergies. The dryness of the weather is what can cause respiratory issues, some foods to consider:

- o Sauerkraut
- o Olives
- o Pickles
- o Leeks
- o Aduki beans
- o Plums
- o Rose hip tea
- o Vinegar
- o Grapes
- o Yogurt
- o Lemon, limes
- o Apples (8)

Water Element: Finally, winter season, when weather turns cold and our core needs warmth. The kidneys represent this element, and when our bodies utilize our storage mechanism. Some foods to consider during this time:

- o Warm hearty soups
- o Whole grains
- o Roasted nuts
- o Dried fruits
- o Small dark beans
- o Seaweeds
- o Steamed winter vegetables (dark greens)
- o Lettuce
- o Watercress
- o Endive
- o Escarole
- o Celery
- o Asparagus
- o Rye, oats, quinoa (8)

It's estimated that diet causes about one third of all cancer cases, almost as many as tobacco. Because cancer is so strongly associated with chronic inflammation, eating foods that fight inflammation can have a chemoprotective effect. According to Deepak Chopra, some cancer prevention foods include lots of fruits and vegetables. Not to mention each food contains more than one cancer preventing chemical. Each hold an abundance of cancer preventing and anti-inflammatory chemicals, such as:

- Carotenoids
- Resveratrol
- Quercitin
- Sulforane (12)

Cancer-fighting chemicals are also found in many teas and spices:

- Green tea
- Turmeric
- Garlic
- Chilies
- Ginger
- Fenugreek
- Fennel
- Clove
- Cinnamon
- Rosemary

"A total of 5,081 patients involved in 50 studies since the 1970s have shown that nutrients do not interfere with conventional cancer treatment. In fact, patients receiving common nutrients like beta-carotene (found in orange pigmented foods like carrots), vitamin D3 (concentrated in egg yolk), vitamins A, B complex, C, E, K, and other food-supplemented antioxidants have fewer side effects, increased therapeutic effectiveness, and higher rates of survival." (16)

There is much more that goes into each of the five elements, I only touched the surface. However, knowing the connection between food, personality traits, emotions, and disease, proves you can take control of your health in a holistic and healing way. Going with the seasons, being aware of the environment you are living in. What foods promote healing during these seasons? Are you being mindful with analyzing your daily symptoms? Eating specific foods to heal and nourish, preparing your meals with mindfulness, symptoms your body is physically manifesting pay attention to as warning signs, you can be cured by approaching a simple holistic approach to your lifestyle.

Dr. David Jockers stated that, antioxidants are also essential for shutting down the communication signals that allow cancer cells to metastasize and destroying cancer stem cells. They also prevent oxidative damage to healthy cells and tissue by supporting detoxification pathways.

Some of the best compounds found in foods that target cancer include:

- **Quercetin:** Antioxidant contained in green tea, red onions, raspberries, and a variety of fruits. Boosts immune response to naturally aid the body in working against cancer cells associated with leukemia, lung, colon, and prostate cancer.

- **Ursolic Acid**: Found in apples and holy basil. Effective against colon, skin, cervical, lung, prostate, and breast cancers.

- **Lycopene**: Rich in tomatoes, grapefruit, and watermelons. Provides protection against cervical, colon, prostate, and lung cancer.

- **Anthocyanins**: Highly concentrated in bilberries, grapes, eggplant, and herbal teas. Suppresses tumors associated with colon cancer and leukemia.

- **Curcumin:** Active component in turmeric. Exhibits powerful chemoprotective activity over numerous cancers such as brain, non-Hodgkin's lymphoma, kidney, and colorectal. (17)

CHAPTER 6

STRESS & MIND-BODY CONNECTION

"All of this is for you. Take it and have gratitude. Give it and feel love."
-Amelia Olson

I am a big proponent of meditation as a part of healing your mind, body, and soul. I find this to always be a journey, connecting not only the mind and body but the soul, who you are deep down. Side note, I was not into meditation in my early teens and twenties, I couldn't sit still, thoughts swirling through my head, until one day after enough practice, I managed to get to this point of complete stillness. I noticed a difference immediately, my neck relaxed, my jaw unclenched, no fear, just being happy and calm. My late teens and early twenties, I was in a mindset of survival and push until you collapse. Which is not beneficial for me anymore, I no longer need to live in a "survival primal" state. I look back and think, "wow, I am a pretty chill person but damn was I internally stressed and always striving for perfection." We create our own worlds based on our limiting beliefs and distorted viewpoints of how we view ourselves. Everyone knows that saying beautiful on the inside, well if you meet someone who is stunning and then they start acting mean to you and others. That shows us, they have insecurities and no self-worth, and we don't really view them as beautiful anymore. How does this all correlate to health?

Meditation helps us to align with ourselves, our true selves, it requires us to sit in stillness. There is a big correlation between a change in your nervous system and mediation in a positive light. If you wake up stressed, your day may end up being… stressed, you go to bed stressed, you wake up stressed. The cycle continues, a great example of this: Let's say you get into an argument with your spouse, this makes you angry (emotion), this is considered your refractory period (part of the brain that processes emotions), instead of dealing with said emotion (punching a pillow, screaming, dancing it out, communicating), you carry that emotion on with you for days. You have now entered a mood, you still repress those emotions, turns into resentment for months which then brings you to eventually a personality trait. Then you say, "oh yeah, I am like this because of this incident that happened seven years ago." How ridiculous does that sound and yet we do this! It does our wellbeing more harm than good.

Dealing with emotions in a healthy way and in a safe environment is the best way to cope. For me, when I was going through my cancer journey as a young adult, I blocked it out of my mind and didn't even dwell on it. At the time, was this what I needed to do? For myself, yes. Did it get me through an extremely emotional and stressful time in my life? Yes. Can I go back and change how I dealt with my emotions? No. So what do I do? I accept it, I had to be **resilient**. I learn from it and do better. Resiliency is KEY to overcoming adversity, there are numerous studies on this, and the affect trauma plays on us after an event. The common theme, how resilient the individual was. This is where I started my journey with meditation.

Mediation and The Brain

The thinking and feeling loop play a big role by turning your thoughts with the exact feelings that matches the thought you are thinking. When you think different thoughts, your brain circuits in corresponding patterns, sequences, and combinations.

This then turns into thoughts, which a network of neurons is activated. The brain produces specific chemicals that match according to your thoughts, in turn creating a feeling. (9)

Knowing this, if you are a person who struggles with negative thoughts daily, living in fear, anxiety, and scarcity. You then turn those negative thoughts into negative emotions, which we know impacts our health negatively. In turn, because you are constantly living out those thoughts and emotions, you will manifest fear and scarcity. So why don't we focus on positive mindset and thoughts? We are conditioned from birth to live up to certain expectations from home life and society, between what you are taught at school, your own trauma, your family, your friends, the media, the list goes on. This creates limiting beliefs, making excuses because of something that happened years ago, "I am angry all of the time because of this incident that happened seven years ago and never got over it." This will set you up for failure and to live a very unfulfilling life. Now knowing this key information, let's think differently, when we do that, we feel differently, when we do that, we act differently. This changes your nervous system to respond differently to the outside world.

"To change is to think greater than how you feel." (9) This means to be greater than the body, no longer in that state of being. When your feelings are now controlling your thoughts, that means your body now has control of your mind. Those "chemicals" created now run the way you unconsciously are wired to react.

"As you unmemorized any emotion that has become a part of your identity, you close the gap between how you appear and who you really are. The side effect of this phenomenon is a release of energy in the form of stored emotion in the body. Once the mind of that emotion is liberated from the body, energy is freed up in the quantum field for you to use as a creator." (9)

Meditation means to become familiar with, aka self-observation. (9) The reason that I personally mediate is because I struggled and somewhat still struggle with fear of being diagnosed with cancer again. I had to unlearn this feeling, an unconscious behavior. I was never a person to mediate in my early adolescence, in terms of what everyone envisions. Sitting crossed legged, not moving and in silence. There are many ways and forms for one to meditate, it is whatever is best for YOU in that moment, in that time.

For me when I was a collegiate athlete, I would practice visualization and breathing techniques. Now in my late twenties, the meaning and way I meditate is different, I sit cross legged, calm, breathing, still and in silence, I usually listen to a guided mediation. It has helped me tremendously, the way I think, act, and feel, it is absolute bliss and joy. The goal is to know who you are, remember and find yourself. You are put on this earth for a specific purpose, part of the game of life is to remember who you are and what your purpose is, what do you bring to the collective to help others. What is your legacy? I no longer view myself as healed because chemotherapy healed me of cancer, no it is because I CHOSE to be cancer free, on a cellular level. Which now brings me to write and share this book with others to get my message across. You can heal yourself; you can live a blissful life, you can have everything you desire, it is a matter of unlearning patterns and behaviors of your past unconscious self so that now your conscious self can do those things naturally.

A great example is from Deepak Chopra, he was interviewed by Tony Robbins, they discussed a study that was conducted with cancer patients who were in a specific protocol to be administered chemotherapy. Half of the research group was given chemotherapy and the other half was given a placebo. The individuals who received the placebo also lost their hair!! Why? It is because they had a belief surrounding chemotherapy and losing your hair, they told themselves they would and so that is what happened.

I am a big fan of Deepak Chopra; he combines his own experience and science, below there are some great findings regarding cancer and healing your own body. "In Ayurveda, a level of total, deep relaxation is the most important precondition for curing any disorder. The underlying concept is that the body knows how to maintain balance unless thrown off by disease; therefore, if one wants to restore the body's own healing ability, everything should be done to bring it back into balance. It is a very simple notion that has profound consequences." (10)

"It is generally agreed that up to 50% of cancer cases are preventable using already-existing knowledge. Everyday lifestyle choices are the main thrust of prevention, which includes not smoking, eating a natural whole-foods diet, avoiding carcinogens in our food, air, and water." (11)

The biggest agreement with all cancer patients and survivors is the fear they go through. The doctors basically giving you a death sentence, when you put that belief into an individual's mind, it will only cause them more harm. It perpetuates the disease. "The fact is that every aged person dies with some malignancy in the body that wasn't the cause of death. In addition, random anomalous or malignant cells are probably present in almost everyone's blood stream. There is no cause for panic over these facts." (13)

Genetics play a factor of course but doctors who treat childhood cancer have raised the success rate from 20% to 80% by targeting specific mutations in the past several decades. The evidence is clear that lifestyle is linked to cancer diagnosis. It accounts for 90% or more of cancer occurrences.(12)

The human brain is truly remarkable and the world's greatest supercomputer. Based off our five senses, every second our brains process billions of data. "It analyzes, examines identifies, extrapolates, classifies, and files information, which it can retrieve for us on an as needed basis." (9) Knowing this information now, why wouldn't you think that you can change or heal yourself? My favorite saying, "if you don't use it, you lose it." This applies for our nerve cells that if not stressed appropriately you lose those firing sequences. However, it also applies that if you continue to learn and stress the nervous system appropriately you can create new neural pathways, including learning, memory, and recovery from brain damage.

Neuroscientists have developed a process known as pruning and sprouting, the learning and unlearning, creating the ability to rise over certain limitations that we have created. (9) The goal is to unify the mind and body to act as one, that is when true change can emerge. We have three brains that take place in this process: "the first brain, the neocortex, the second brain, is the limbic or emotional brain, responsible for creating, maintaining, and organizing chemicals in the body. The third brain, the cerebellum, is the seat of the subconscious mind." (9)

Meditation allows us to change our brain, body, and state of being, without taking physical action or interaction with the external environment. We enter the subconscious mind which is 95% of our everyday habits and motor control. (9) The goal is to work on our internal environment, bringing inner peace, harmony, joy, compassion, content, happiness, all emotions that positively influence our state of being (mind-body connection). The act of living in and being whatever, it is you what to be, for the sake of this book, let's say you want to be healthy and cancer free. You must envision yourself in that current state of being, healthy and happy, what would you be doing, what would you look like, how would you be acting, what are the feelings that come up?

This is where meditation takes us, into that state of being, that calm and still place, as if it were already happening, our minds do not know the difference between a scenario we create in our head based off emotions or the outside reality (read that again). The power we hold we as human beings and we don't even realize; we must heal ourselves internally first.

"Get in your head, you're dead" -Tony Robbins

Other modalities of healing and minimizing stress and fear daily:

- Frequency Sound Healing (this is a favorite of mine)

I personally use this modality for healing (to an extent), whether it be a headache or going through stress. I will literally go on YouTube and type in "frequency sound healing for …" Each sound has a different type of hertz that brings your body into a healing state naturally. You can also go to specific classes held at yoga studios or holistic practices. It is meant to bring you back to homeostasis and give your body the green light to go head and start the healing process. I predict that treatment rooms for pediatric patients will change drastically. Where they utilize a room with the specific sound frequency hertz to destroy cancer cells (which is between 100,000 and 300,000 hertz), there will be coloring and laughing, and it will be a pleasant place to heal. Which brought me to learn about Vibroacoustic, this modality can help individuals recognize a deep state of relaxation, it changes your nervous system to be predominantly in a parasympathetic state (which is where the subconscious mind lives), all through frequency waves and music. Notice how mediation and sound frequency healing change the state of your nervous system to become less charged and promote healing.

According to the National Institute of Health, since 1995, they run the most extensive program in the U.S. for vibroacoustic pain and symptom reduction, treating over 50,000 patients per year. In one study, Dr. George Patrick measured the physiological and behavioral effectiveness of these interventions with 272 patients and found over 50% reduction of pain and symptoms. In his findings he concluded that pain relief is induced by relaxation. The body using the vibrations and frequencies through music as a self-healing tool. Another study done at the Jupiter Medical Center in Florida, has shown tests done with chemotherapy patients. There was a 62.8% reduction of anxiety and 61.6% reduction of fatigue for 27 patients in 41 vibroacoustic sessions. (14)

What happens exactly in the mind and body during these sessions?

- Slows down the heart rate
- Decreases blood pressure
- Clears the mind from being in survival mode
- Creates calmness by enhancing the parasympathetic nervous system
- Relaxes the mind and body
- Changes your brain waves to become slower
- Creates homeostasis in the body = healing

It is so fascinating that music and sound frequency can heal the body and alter our physiology. Soothing music provides a deep state of relaxation, which I mentioned prior activates your parasympathetic nervous system (best to be in this state majority of life unless in a life altering situation or danger). Based off those healing frequency waves it can help optimize your autonomic, immune, endocrine, and neuropeptide systems. It also helps to reduce anxiety and fear. Responses have been linked to the function of the brain, music being a catalyst to enhance our own learning abilities and self- healing. (14)

International studies have been done and can attest to the effectiveness of Vibroacoustic Therapy for treatments of cancer, cardiovascular disease, hypertension, migraine headaches, gastrointestinal ulcers, Raynaud's disease, Parkinson's, fibromyalgia, polyarthritis, sports injury, low back pain, neck and shoulder pain, autism, insomnia, depression, and anxiety disorders. Not to mention the work of Dr. Joe Dispenza, also supports this research in his books and his own findings working with mediation, frequency sound healing, and breathing exercises.

This information is huge for us to understand and be open minded to. These findings show that there is hope for different treatment for illness, disease, and injury. A non-toxic, non-invasive, and effective way to heal yourself. Science and music seem to be merging for healing and new treatment therapies and protocols. I don't know about you but that makes me EXCITED. This should give you all so much joy, faith, and hope. Treatment rooms I believe will be looking very different for pediatric patients especially, utilizing sound frequency as a healing modality.

Other modalities for managing/healing stress, anxiety, and more:

- Breathing techniques
- Sports
- Nature
- Painting
- Walking your pet
- Laughing
- Seeking a licensed therapist or support group
- Acupuncture, massage, cupping
- Praying
- Yoga
- Dancing
- Singing
- Writing
- Reading
- Lots of activities you enjoy bringing you into the present moment
- Aromatherapy

There are five essential oils that contain anti-cancer properties:

1) **Frankincense:** anti-inflammatory, anti-cancer properties, boost immune system, reduces stress, pain reliver.

2) **Lavender:** supports cancer healing, anti-tumoral, inhibits cell growth, antibacterial, relaxation.

3) **Myrrh:** anti-inflammatory properties, healthy hormone balance, pain reliever, anti-fungal.

4) **Peppermint:** reveals antioxidant and cancer inhibiting properties, suppress growth of tumors, antiangiogenic properties, antiseptic, antimicrobial components.

5) **Turmeric (curcumin):** found to inhibit enzymes like COX-2 that cause inflammation which can lead to cancer, cuts cancer cells off their fuels and oxygen source, stops the spread of cancer cells, promotes cell death of cancer cells and many more beneficial properties. (16)

- Travel
- Spirituality
- Social Media fasting
- Not watching the news or mainstream media
- Self- love and self-care
- Family time
- Love and compassion
- Giving back to others and society
- Community

CHAPTER 7

THE JOURNEY CONTINUES, NOW WHAT?

"Live as if everything is rigged in your favor"
-Rumi

I know we have covered a lot of information; your head may even be spinning. It is okay. My point I really want to get across is being able to accept the challenges and adversities we face in life, know every single person has them, be **resilient**. However, we don't give ourselves enough credit, we need to show ourselves some love. I look back and think how hard I was on myself, and knowing this information discussed in this book, did I do it to myself? Who knows, maybe. The world you create internally is what drives your external world. That worry, that fear, that anxiety, which by the way is one of the top leading causes of death. The best thing to do is have faith, trust, and let go. WAY easier said than done. What I do know is that I cannot dwell on the past and think why me. The victim mentality is not for me, and it shouldn't be for you either. You should not fear death, it is a part of life, do not live your life in fear ever.

I decided to be proactive about my healing journey, writing this book is part of it. Each developmental stage I go through, new feelings and emotions emerge, and new healing takes place. In March 2020, seven years later after my thyroid surgery, I was told by my doctor at Memorial Sloane Kettering, that they found two suspicious spots in my neck, one on the left side (which that part of the thyroid was removed in the prior surgery seven years ago), it was a lymph node and one nodule on the right side where the rest of my thyroid lives. When I tell you I had a mental breakdown after finding that news out, but this is what I told myself, "I don't have cancer and I am not getting another surgery, it is not an option for me." I was and am resilient.

As I waited in the lobby of Memorial Sloane Kettering for another biopsy and ultrasound, I couldn't help but look around and just observe how much worse the other patients were in there. I felt a sense of compassion and hope, solidifying this would not be me. As I went into the ultrasound room, I sat down, and I could feel my heart beating out of my chest and sweat started to drip down my face. I started to get triggered, my breath was short and shallow, as the ultrasound and biopsy are happening, I tried my best to remain cool (I literally had a needle going into my neck). Once the nurse and doctor were done, I broke down into tears and had a full-on panic attack in the room (I don't ever suffer from these). The fear started to kick in, the doubt, the what if. I continued this breakdown in the car not knowing what the outcome would be. I called my mom and my best friend; they always help me and calmed me down from going off a mental cliff. Both knew that everything would be okay.

After this incident, my lab results took over four weeks to get back. Then another week just to get the results from my doctor. The mental toughness, focus, hope and spiritual journey that I had to have during that time frame was enduring to say the very least. Like we spoke about in the previous chapters, fear and anxiety can create a downward spiral in health, mentally and physically. When I FINALLY received the results my doctor says, "well we have good news mostly, good news the left side lymph node is nothing, the right side where the nodule is located well the results came back inconclusive." I pondered what he said for a minute and replied, "this is all great news, I don't have cancer."

He then said, "we now have two options, we can either keep doing the ultrasounds every six months for the next two years or we can do surgery to remove the other side of the thyroid." I am the type of person that when I am given options, especially regarding my health, the answer just comes to me, I have a gut reaction and I just know. I laughed and said, "I'll take the ultrasound every six months for $1,000 please." He agreed and told me that if I was his daughter, he would suggest the same thing. Instantly a relief came over me, I knew and told myself I would never have cancer again. I can sit here and happily say that I have received another ultrasound and testing since then and there has been no change in growth and I am healthy and cancer free.

That moment and waiting period is what truly tested me and brought me on this healing journey today and that I share with you all. Letting go, knowing, and being proactive is what got me here today. After that it led me to reading the book, *Winning the War On Cancer,* by Sylvie Beljanski, and I will never look at cancer the same again. I took a deep dive into holistic medicine and started taking the natural supplements suggested by The Beljanski Foundation. I live my life according to how I want to live my life, no one is going to tell me otherwise. I hope whoever reads this book is inspired to change their life for the better and take ownership of their health. Self-love and compassion seem to be the driving force and something we all need to work on. Remember when you can fill up your own cup, you can give to others, creating a positive ripple effect within the collective.

I had been taking those supplements and following a specific protocol from The Beljanski Foundation *(Pao Pereira)* for two months prior to my most recent ultrasound and checkup. During the ultrasound the technician who I hadn't seen in just about six or seven years and did my first ultrasound ever, stated that the lymph node on the left side where they originally were concerned about looked smaller, but she didn't know if she was seeing things. I sat there and paused for a second and asked her to repeat herself. I did not mention to her I was taking *Pao Pereira.* Which by the way is on the Memorial Sloane Kettering website for healing, with minimal information and pretty much hidden. I then told her I was taking the supplement and her jaw dropped (she was shocked I even knew about it). That solidified to me that these supplements work, and all would be well.

I received hope reading this article from Deepak Chopra, he discusses the power of fear and what it does to people. If you believe it and you think it, you are setting the tone for your life and outcome, there is a greater chance it can happen. It is hopeful moving forward because according to the American Cancer Society, in 2017, the overall cancer deaths declined by 25%. To quote the ACA's website, "During the most recent decade of available data, the rate of new cancer diagnoses decreased by about 2% per year in men and stayed about the same in women. The cancer death rate declined by about 1.5% annually in both men and women." (11)

Fear & Well-Being

Fear and love cannot co-exist without the other. Fear can be crippling and literally sucks the life out of your soul. This diminishes your wellbeing and when you are not showing up for yourself you cannot show up for anyone else. We can turn on this fight or flight mode due to fears and survival mode, by a thought alone. This is where the conditioned self, the program, the survival primal state of you shows up. We are conditioned to be living in fear from birth, thanks to society, media, and our norms. When you are putting your faith into another human being like they are God and not equal to you, you are less than, this is where you steer off the path of you true self.

Love heals all, this cures fear, this allows you to be your true self, filling up your cup, feeding your soul and then you can show up for others and especially yourself. It can create miracles, including curing yourself of illness, yes even cancer. There are countless near-death experiences told by others who have come out and shared their stories. The underlying theme and message are to live your life the way you want to live your life, through love and being aware of thy self, being in the present moment, laughing a lot, self-love, living out your purpose and serving others. Aligning with yourself, it takes time, but once you cross over, know you will never look back, that's how good it is.

A story from Dr. Joe Dispenza and his book *Breaking the Habit of Being Yourself,* "Bill, 57, was a roofing contractor. A lesion had appeared on his face, his dermatologist diagnosed him with malignant melanoma. Bill underwent, surgeries, radiation, and chemotherapy. Yet the cancer kept showing up on other body parts and organs. Bill experienced, naturally, "Why me?" moments. He clung onto the unfairness of other co-workers being exposed to the sun like himself and them being fine. After more treatment, in a moment, he went into self-reflection and wondered if his own thoughts, emotions and actions were making him sick. He realized for more than 30 years he had been stuck in resentment, feeling he always had to give up for what he wanted for the sake of others. He had a victim mentality. His state of being had signaled the same gene for so long that they had created the disease. Bill decided to change his ways, he left his familiar environment and went on a retreat to Mexico. For five mornings, he became an observer of his thoughts and feelings, he then paid attention to his previously unconscious behaviors and actions. He decided to halt any thought, behavior or emotion that was unloving toward himself. Next, he decided to think about the new self he would be. He needed to think, act, and feel his new self. Shortly after he returned, the tumor on Bill's calf fell off, a week later he went to the doctor, and he was cancer free. He has remained that way. By firing his brain in new ways, Bill changed biologically and chemically from his previous self. As a result, he signaled new genes in new ways, and those cancer cells couldn't coexist with his new mind, new internal chemistry, and new self." (9)

I believe that a huge contributor to this global epidemic of illness and disease (besides environment, water, food, and products) is lack of self-identity and self-love. The best example I have of this is about Pluto. Yes, the planet, whatever you want to consider it as. Pluto doesn't give a shit if you think it is a star or planet because Pluto is too busy doing Pluto things, like revolving. Pluto doesn't give a damn, there are more important things to be accomplished and neither should you. Who cares what anyone else thinks about you, because guess what the only thing that matters is what you think about you. What is most important is you can take care of yourself, nurture yourself and live out your purpose in this life.

No one seems to realize their true potential, true self, and that their brain is a supercomputer that can change your thoughts in an instant, faster than a millisecond. The power that you hold as an individual is so insane. We apparently can't fathom this information and so we are like, "yeah, whatever, it is easier to play this role of a victim instead and live-in fear." Let's talk about the identity gap, this is the gap between who we really are and how we appear. How we appear: the identity I project to the outer environment, who I want you to think I am, the façade, ideal for the world. Who we really are: how I feel, who I really am, how I am on the inside, ideal for self. (9)

"When we memorize addictive emotional states such as guilt, shame, fear, anxiety, judgement, depression, self-importance, or hatred, we develop a gap between *the way we appear and the way we really are.*" (9) This gap varies from person to person, it depends on past life experiences, throughout different points in our lives, the bigger the gap the more addicted to our emotions we memorize.

If you take away only this bit of the above paragraph out of this whole book, then my job is complete. That is how important about knowing what fear does to our mind, body, and soul. Don't do any of the things I have spoken about in previous chapters out of fear for your health or of what society/groups think of you. Do it for yourself, do it because that's your damn birth right, do it because you know it will feel good to live true to thy self. Why live-in fear? What fun is that? Life is supposed to be enjoyable, through human experience, you can create heaven on earth with your thoughts alone. Do it because you love yourself enough to act on it, not because of fear of the future, what any group or persons says, and what if.

My healing and spiritual journey won't stop, and it will continue to evolve, and I will continue to inspire, learn, and educate. Learning about myself, what works best for me, how to heal naturally, research, educate and most importantly give back to my fellow cancer fighters and survivors. I was nominated for Leukemia and Lymphoma Society, Woman of the Year 2021 Long Island, again such a full circle moment. Getting involved in the cancer community has healed me in so many ways, I can't even describe. I am a certified "Imerman Angel" Mentor Angel where I can support fellow fighter and or cancer survivors through the emotional aspect of their journey. Knowing that I can and will make a difference, giving others light and hope to keep fighting for themselves. Making so many new friends and connections, being a part of a young adult community of cancer fighters and survivors, has accelerated my part in this world to give back. Now I can share this with all of you, what I have learned, endured, and hope to give you faith. You do not need to do this all on your own, be proactive, live your life to the fullest, do what you love and fulfill your purpose here on earth.

"The only way to have a friend is to be one."
-Stephanie Bradshaw

Take Away:

- Laugh always
- Give back
- Move everyday
- Meditate often (whatever that means to you)
- Train the way you think, act, and move daily
- Be who you want to be
- Do not live-in fear, live in love
- Accomplish what you want to accomplish
- Be kind to yourself, self-love is the key
- Your beliefs set the tone for your life and what you desire
- The internal world you create vibrates and creates your external world

Cancer Communities, Organizations, Non-Profits, and Foundations:

The Beljanski Foundation
The Truth About Cancer
St. Jude Children's Research Hospital
The Leukemia and Lymphoma Society
The MaxLove Foundation

Cohen's Children's Medical Foundation
Stupid Cancer
Team in Training
Big Climb
Imerman Angels
The Luna Foundation

REFERENCES & RESOURCES

1) Beljanski, Sylvie, "Winning The War On Cancer: The Epic Journey Towards A Natural Cure," pg. 1, 2, 3, 15, 25, 109, 121, 146

2) Cabano, Catherine, In On Around You, "Clean Beauty Checklist," 2021, pg. 8

3) Gena Bradshaw and Erica Suter, "Girls to Queens Podcast, The 7 Gems of Mastery," 2021, https://podcasts.apple.com/us/podcast/episode-2-the-7-gems-to-live-your-best-life/id1573946392?i=1000527583232

4) Bradshaw Personal Fitness, "The Growing Crisis of Chronic Disease," 2021, https://bpfit.com/the-growing-crisis-of-chronic-disease/

5) Reiner et al. BMC Public Health 2013, 13:813 http://www.biomedcentral.com/1471-2458/13/813)

6) Ashcraft KA, et al. Exercise as adjunct therapy in cancer. Seminars in Radiation Oncology. 2018;29:16.https://www.mayoclinic.org/diseases-conditions/cancer/in-depth/secret-weapon-during-cancer-treatment-exercise/art-20457584

7) Schroeder EC, Franke WD, Sharp RL, Lee D-c (2019) Comparative effectiveness of aerobic, resistance, and combined training on cardiovascular disease risk

factors: A randomized controlled trial. PLoS ONE 14(1): e0210292. https://doi.org/10.1371/journal.pone.0210292 https://journals.plos.org/plosone/article?id=10.1371/journal.pone.0210292

8) Paul Pitchford, "Healing With Whole Foods: Asian Traditions and Modern Nutrition," 3rd edition, pg. 1, 2, 8, 305, 317, 332, 337, 346, 354

9) Dr. Joe Dispenza, "Breaking the Habit of Being Yourself, How to Lose Your Mind and Create A New One," 2017, pg. 57, 108, 124, 150, 167

10) Deepak Chopra, M.D., "Quantum Healing, Exploring the Frontiers of Mind/Body Medicine," 2015 https://www.penguinrandomhouse.ca/books/27394/quantum-healing-revised-and-updated-by-deepak-chopra/9781101884973/excerpt

11) Deepak Chopra, M.D. and Rudolph E. Tanzi, Ph.D, "Optimistic Thoughts About Cancer- For Real," July 13th, 2017 https://choprafoundation.org/articles/optimistic-thoughts-about-cancer-for-real/

12) Deepak Chopra, M.D. ," Cancer A Preventable Disease is Creating A Revolution," August 12 2012, https://www.deepakchopra.com/articles/cancer-a-preventable-disease-is-creating-a-revolution/)

13) Deepak Chopra, M.D., "Cancer Prevention How mind Body and Meditation Creates Optimism," August 21st, 2017, https://chopra.com/articles/cancer-prevention-how-mind-body-and-medicine-creates-optimism

14) https://www.naturalresonancecenter.com/research/

15) Anand, P., Kunnumakkara, A. B., Sundaram, C., Harikumar, K. B., Tharakan, S. T., Lai, O. S., Sung, B., & Aggarwal, B. B. (2008). Cancer is a preventable disease that requires major lifestyle changes. *Pharmaceutical research*, *25*(9), 2097–2116. https://doi.org/10.1007/s11095-008-9661-9

16) Ty Bollinger, "5 Cancer-Fighting Essential Oils & 5 Ways to Use Them," June 8th, 2021, https://thetruthaboutcancer.com/essential-oils-for-cancer/

17) Dr. David Jockers DC, MS, CSCS, "7 Ways Nutritional Therapy Works Against Cancer," April 10th, 2021, https://thetruthaboutcancer.com/nutritional-therapy-cancer/

18) Dr. Joe Dispenza, "Becoming Supernatural, How Common People Are Doing the Uncommon," 2017, pg. 47

Printed in the United States
by Baker & Taylor Publisher Services